1

Table of Contents

PREVIEW

The lymphatic system is a network of tissues, vessels and organs that work together to move a colorless, watery fluid called lymph back into your circulatory system (your bloodstream).

Some 20 liters of plasma flow through your body's arteries and smaller arteriole blood vessels and capillaries every day. After delivering nutrients to the body's cells and tissues and receiving their waste products, about 17 liters are returned to the circulation by way of veins. The remaining three liters seep through the capillaries and into your body's tissues. The lymphatic system collects this excess fluid, now called lymph, from tissues in your body and moves it along until it's ultimately returned to your bloodstream.

Your lymphatic system has many functions. Its key functions include:

Maintains fluid levels in your body: As just described, the lymphatic system collects excess fluid that drains from cells and tissue throughout your body and returns it to your bloodstream, which is then recirculated through your body.

Absorbs fats from the digestive tract: Lymph includes fluids from your intestines that contain fats and proteins and transports it back to your bloodstream.

Protects your body against foreign invaders: The lymphatic system is part of the immune system. It produces and releases lymphocytes (white blood cells) and other immune cells that monitor and then destroy the foreign invaders — such as bacteria, viruses, parasites and fungi — that may enter your body.

LYMPHATIC DIET RECIPES

BREAKFAST

1. Comforting Winter Breakfast Porridge

Prep Time: 45 minutes

Cook Time: 1 hour

Yield: servings 6

Ingredients

For the Porridge:

- 2 tablespoons chia seeds
- 1 cup plus 6 tablespoons almond milk or coconut milk, divided
- 3 cups purified water
- 1/2 cup pearled barley, rinsed in a strainer
- Sea salt
- 1 tablespoon coconut sugar
- 1 teaspoon vanilla extract (optional)
- 1-1/2 teaspoons ghee (optional)

For the Candied Kumquats:

- 3/4 cup honey
- 1/2 cup purified water
- 1 vanilla bean, seeds scraped out
- 2 pints (about 4 cups) kumquats, sliced

Instructions

1. Combine the chia seeds and 6 tablespoons of the almond milk or coconut milk in a small bowl and whisk until well mixed to prevent clumping.
2. Set aside.
3. Bring the water to a boil in a medium saucepan. Add the barley and salt, to taste, lower the heat to a strong simmer, and cook for 30 minutes, partially covered.
4. Check and stir periodically to make sure that not all the water has evaporated, and to prevent the barley from sticking to the bottom of the pan.
5. Add the remaining 1 cup of almond milk, the coconut sugar, and the vanilla, if using, to the barley.
6. Bring the mixture back to a slow simmer and cook for another 10 minutes, uncovered and stirring periodically, until the barley is fully cooked and most of the liquid is absorbed.

7. Taste and adjust with more salt as needed. Add the ghee, if using, and stir to incorporate.

8. Stir in the soaked chia seeds and remove the pan from the heat.

9. Distribute among individual bowls, add more milk and/or ghee, if preferred, and top with Candied Kumquats.

10. To Prepare the Kumquats

11. In a medium saucepan over medium heat, combine the honey, water, and vanilla bean seeds and pod.

12. Bring to a gentle boil. Add in the kumquats and bring the mixture back to a boil, then lower the heat and simmer for 10 minutes until syrupy.

13. Remove the pan from the heat and let the kumquats cool in the syrup.

14. Store the candied kumquats in an airtight container in the refrigerator for up to 1 week.

Prep Time: 30 minutes

Cook Time: 1 hour

Yield: servings 30 small cookies

Ingredients

- 1 cup (2 sticks) unsalted butter, softened
- 1/2 cup granulated sugar
- 2 large eggs
- 1 teaspoon pure mint extract
- 1/2 cup unsweetened, alkalized cocoa powder
- 2 cups sifted all-purpose flour
- About 2 tablespoons all-purpose flour, for dusting work surface
- 2 to 4 tablespoons granulated sugar, for sprinkling on cookie tops
- About 4 ounces semisweet chocolate, melted
- White Chocolate-Mint Mousse:
- 1/2 cup loosely packed mint leaves, stems removed, coarsely chopped
- 1 cup heavy cream, divided
- 6 ounces white chocolate, finely chopped

Instructions

1. To make mousse, place mint and 1/2 cup cream in saucepan and bring to scalding over medium heat. Turn off heat. Steep about 30 minutes. Strain cream mixture into another clean saucepan, pressing excess liquid from mint. Add chopped white chocolate to cream and place over low heat. Stir constantly just until chocolate is melted and mixture is very smooth. Transfer to medium bowl. Cover surface flush with plastic wrap and allow to cool to room temperature, about 40 minutes. Using an electric mixer with whip attachment, whip remaining cream to stiff peaks. Fold into chocolate mixture. Chill mousse 3 to 4 hours or until thick and creamy.

2. To make cookies, place butter and 1/2 cup sugar in electric mixer with paddle attachment. Cream until well blended, about 2 minutes. Add eggs one at a time, beating well after each addition. Scrape down sides of bowl. Continue to beat at high speed until light and fluffy, another 2 to 3 minutes. Stir in mint extract. Stir together cocoa powder and flour and combine with butter mixture, stirring just until evenly blended. Divide dough, shape into two disks and wrap each tightly in plastic wrap. Chill at least 4 hours or until

dough is firm to touch. Meanwhile, with rack in center of oven, preheat to 350 degrees. Line two cookie sheets with parchment paper and set aside. On lightly floured work surface, roll out one disk of dough to about 1/8-inch thickness. Cut with 1 1/2-inch fluted round cookie cutter and transfer rounds to cookie sheet. Using 1/2-inch heart-shaped cookie cutter, cut a window in half of the cookies. These will become sandwich tops. Sprinkle evenly with granulated sugar. Bake 12 to 14 minutes, or until cookies are firm and lightly browned on bottoms. Remove to racks to cool. Repeat with second half of dough. Allow cookies to cool completely. Using a small knife, spread thin layer of melted chocolate on bottoms of windowless cookies and place cookie chocolate side up. Let chocolate set.

3. To assemble sandwiches, fit pastry bag with #10 round tip and fill halfway with mousse. Pipe small amount of mousse on top of set chocolate. Place cookie with window, right side-up, on top of mousse. Press gently to squeeze mousse to edges. Store unfilled cookies in airtight containers up to a week at room temperature. Filled cookies should be refrigerated, and are best served within 24 hours.

Prep Time: 50 minutes

Cook Time: 1 hour 30 Minutes

Yield: servings 4

Ingredient

- 1 eggplant, sliced
- 1 red onion, sliced
- 1 zucchini, sliced
- 2 tomatoes, sliced
- 3 tbsp. ghee or fat of choice
- 1 tsp. sea salt
- 1/2 tsp. fresh cracked pepper
- Handful of fresh thyme, stripped off ste

Instructions

1. Preheat the oven to 425 degrees Fahrenheit. Place the vegetables in a big bowl, and drizzle with the fat. Add the sea salt, pepper, thyme, and garlic. Using a large spoon, gently toss to coat. In a round, well-greased baking dish, place the vegetable slices in a repeating

pattern of concentric circles. You can also use a
rectangular dish, and make a pattern of alternating
rows. Add a bit more ghee on top of the vegetables,
and cover with foil. Cook for 20 minutes, remove the
foil, and baste the vegetables with the juices in the
bottom of the pan. Cook for an additional 20 minutes,
basting once again halfway through. Remove from the
oven and serve.

Prep Time: 50 minutes

Cook Time: 1 hour 30 Minutes

Yield: servings 4

Ingredient

- 1 pound chorizo sausage
- 2 potatoes, diced
- 1 red bell pepper, sliced
- 1 orange bell pepper, sliced
- 8 ounces Cotija cheese, crumbled
- Salsa
- 8 to 10 tortillas
- Camp stove or campfire coals
- Skillet or Dutch ove

Instructions

1. Crumble sausage and cook for about 10 minutes over medium-high heat with the diced potato until sausage is brown and potato is soft. Add bell pepper slices,

cooking until soft. Top with crumbled Cotija cheese and set aside, keeping warm.

2. Warm each tortilla briefly in the skillet and fill with meat mixture and salsa as desired.

Prep Time: 10 minutes

Cook Time: 30 Minutes

Yield: servings 4

Ingredient

- 1 refrigerated pie crust (or 1 package pie crust mix prepared according to directions)
- 8 slices cooked bacon, crumbled
- 1 cup shredded cheddar cheese
- 1 1/2 cups milk
- 1/2 cup all purpose flour
- 1 teaspoon salt
- 2 green onions, finely diced
- 1 tablespoon fresh or dried parsley
- 8 eggs, beaten
- Ketchup or salsa

Equipment

- Parchment paper
- Charcoal briquettes or campfire coals
- 10-inch Dutch oven

- 8 coals on bottom
- 14 coals on top, 350 degrees

Instructions

1. Line the bottom of a 10-inch Dutch oven with strips of folded baking parchment up the side of the oven to aid in removing the pie. Unroll the pie crust and place in the bottom of the oven, stretching up the sides. Pinch edges between thumb and forefinger to scallop.
2. Sprinkle bacon and cheese on the bottom of the pie crust. Add milk, flour, salt, green onions and parsley to the beaten eggs and mix well. Pour egg mixture into the pie crust.
3. Cover and bake with heat on top and bottom for 45 minutes until eggs are set. Allow cooling for 10 minutes before lifting out the pie. Serve with ketchup or salsa.

Prep Time: 10 minutes

Cook Time: 30 Minutes

Yield: servings 6

Ingredient

- 2 cups spelt flakes
- 1 cup old-fashioned rolled oats
- ½ cup bran flakes
- 2/3 cup chopped almonds
- 1/3 cup sesame seeds
- ½ cup sunflower seeds
- ¼ cup chopped walnuts
- ½ cup honey
- 2 teaspoons ground cinnamon
- 1 teaspoon ground ginger
- 1 teaspoon ground ginseng, optional
- ½ cup chopped dried apricots• ½ cup raisins
- ½ cup dried cranberries
- Use 3 cups rolled oats in total if spelt flakes are not available.

Instructions

1. Preheat oven to 375 degrees. Lightly oil two rimmed baking sheets.

2. On one prepared baking sheet, spread spelt, oats and bran. On other sheet, spread almonds, sesame seeds, sunflower seeds and walnuts. Stagger sheets in oven and toast for 8 minutes.

3. Remove sheet with nuts and seeds from oven and cool. Stir grains on the remaining sheet and continue toasting for another 6 to 8 minutes, or until lightly browned.

4. Meanwhile, in a small saucepan, heat honey, cinnamon, ginger and ginseng (if using) until just simmering. Remove from heat.

5. Remove grains from oven and transfer to a large bowl. Stir in toasted nuts. Drizzle warm honey mixture over contents. Add apricots, raisins and cranberries; stir lightly to mix. Cool. Store in an airtight container in refrigerator up to 2 months

Prep Time: 25 minutes

Cook Time: 40 Minutes

Yield: servings 1

Ingredient

- 1 teaspoon cooking oil, preferably rosemary flavored
- 3 large eggs
- 1/8 teaspoon salt
- Freshly ground black pepper to taste
- 2 tablespoons shredded Jarlsberg or ¬imported Gruyère cheese
- 2 tablespoons snipped chives
- 3 tablespoons julienne-sliced sorrel

Instructions

1. With a soft paper towel, film a 7-inch or larger nonstick omelet pan with the oil. Heat the pan over medium-high heat while you whisk the eggs, salt, and pepper in a bowl with a fork.
2. Pour the eggs into the pan in a thin layer.

3. Holding the pan handle in one hand and the spatula in the other, tilt the pan slightly while you push the spatula from the lower right side of the pan all the way through the omelet to the upper left, pushing the cooked eggs off the bottom of the pan and letting the uncooked portion flow around the spatula. Flatten the omelet, poking it gent¬ly with the tip of the spatula. Now tilt the pan the other way and push the spatula from the upper right through to the lower left to make an X; flatten again.

4. Sprinkle on the cheese and cook a few seconds longer.

5. When the omelet is nearly done, toss on the sorrel and chives, fold the omelet in half, and slide it onto a warm plate.

Prep Time: 55 minutes

Cook Time: 60 Minutes

Yield: servings 1

Ingredient

- 1 tsp coconut oil
- 1/2 tsp mustard seeds
- 2-3 curry leaves
- Snake gourd – Cut and chopped into small pieces (Try to get locally grown organic snake gourd)
- 1 carrot, chopped
- 2 tbsp grated coconut
- 1/4 tsp turmeric
- 1/2 tsp cumin seeds
- 1/2 tsp chili powder
- Salt – to taste

Instructions

1. Wash and chop off the top and bottom of snake gourd and cut it into small pieces. Heat oil in a small pan

and when hot splutter mustard seeds. Add chopped snake gourd, Carrots, turmeric powder, and mix well. Add 1/2 cup water. Let it cook without lid on low-medium heat for 20-25 minutes. Stir occasionally and continue cooking until the vegetables are tender. Now, in a blender add scraped coconut, cumin seeds and chili powder. Crush it and add with cooked vegetables. Add salt to taste. Serve warm with rice.

2. Instead of snake gourd you can use French beans, beets, cabbage, or your choice of vegetable. Make sure you add the right amount of water to cook the vegetable.

3. Ladies Finger (Okra) Stir Fry

Ingredient

- 1/2 c washed and cut okra
- 1 tsp coconut oil
- 1/2 tsp mustard seeds
- 2-3 curry leaves
- Salt to taste
- 1/2 tsp pepper powder

Instructions

1. In a sauce pan, add one tsp. coconut oil. When hot, add mustard seeds and curry leaves. When mustard seed splutters add the cut okra. Sauté okra well and cover and cook in medium flame for 2-3 minutes. Now add the required amount of salt and pepper powder. Cook for 5 more minutes without lid. Serve with warm rice.

2. Fish Gravy

3. Here I have used tuna fish (fresh and organic) due to its impressive nutritional benefits. Tuna fish is rich in omega-3 fatty acids, vitamins. Proteins and minerals. Of course, it is delicious as well.

Ingredient

- 1/2 c shallots, chopped
- 1 tsp ginger-garlic paste
- 1/2 c tuna fish, cleaned and chopped to small pieces
- 1 tsp chili powder
- 1/2 tsp tamarind paste
- 2-3 curry leaves
- 1/2 tsp turmeric powder
- 1 tsp coconut oil
- 1/4 tsp fenugreek seeds

- 1/2 tsp mustard seeds
- Salt to taste
- 1 tomato, sliced

Instructions

1. Heat oil in a sauce pan. When oil is hot, add the curry leaves, mustard seeds and fenugreek. When mustard seeds splutter add in the shallots. Sauté well. When the color turns light brown to golden add ginger garlic paste, turmeric, and sliced tomatoes. Mix well. Cover and cook for 5-7 minutes. When tomato is fully mashed and cooked add chili powder and mix well. Now, add ½ cup of warm water and tuna fish. Add tamarind paste and cook until tuna fish is well cooked. Serve warm with rice.

2. Variations: This is a spicy dish. You can alter the quantity of chili powder or even add 1/4 cup of coconut milk in the end to reduce spiciness. If you are vegan replace tuna fish with cooked black eyes peas and follow all other steps.

Prep Time: 28 minutes

Cook Time: 50 Minutes

Yield: servings 6

Ingredient

- 7 organic eggs
- 2 tablespoons water
- 3 tablespoons fresh parsley, minced
- 3 scallions, finely minced
- 1/4 teaspoon sea salt
- 1/4 teaspoon black pepper
- 1 orange bell pepper, diced
- 7 spears asparagus, diced
- 1 clove garlic, finely minced
- 1 tablespoon extra-virgin olive oil
- 1 Roma tomato, diced
- 1/2 cup freshly grated Romano or Parmesan cheese

Instructions

1. In a mixing bowl, whisk together eggs, water, parsley, scallions, salt, and pepper. Set aside.

2. Preheat oven to 375 degrees Fahrenheit.

3. Heat an oven-safe sauté pan on the stove over medium heat. Sauté bell pepper, asparagus, and garlic in olive oil until softened, 2 to 3 minutes.

4. Reduce heat to medium-low and pour egg mixture into the pan. Occasionally stir eggs gently, tilting the pan to allow the uncooked eggs to run toward the edges until the eggs begin to set.

5. Sprinkle the tomatoes and cheese over the eggs. Bake until puffed and golden, approximately 10 to 12 minutes.

6. Slice frittata into 6 wedges. Garnish with additional parsley, if desired.

Prep Time: 28 minutes

Cook Time: 50 Minutes

Yield: servings 6

Ingredient

- 3/4 cup unbleached flour
- 1/4 cup whole-wheat flour
- 1 tablespoon ground flaxseed
- 2 teaspoons baking powder
- 1/2 cup granulated sugar
- Pinch of salt
- 1/2 cup sea buckthorn berries, fresh or frozen
- 1 egg, beaten
- 1/4 cup butter, melted
- 1/2 cup milk

Instructions

1. Preheat oven to 350 degrees Fahrenheit. Place parchment liners in a 12-cup muffin pan.

2. Mix together flours, flaxseed, baking powder, sugar, and salt in a medium bowl. Add sea buckthorn berries, and mix to coat. Make a well in the center; set aside.

3. In a small bowl, mix together egg, butter, and milk. Pour mixture into well in dry ingredients, and stir until just combined.

4. Divide batter evenly among cups in prepared muffin pan. Bake for 15 minutes, or until a toothpick inserted in the center comes out clean.

5. Optional Dietary Substitutions:

6. To make flax gel to substitute for 1 egg, combine 1 tablespoon ground flaxseed with 3 tablespoons warm water. Let stand for 5 minutes, then use as directed in the recipe.

7. Replace the milk with almond or cashew milk.

8. Margarine (either dairy or nondairy) may be used instead of the butter.

9. A gluten-free flour blend can be substituted cup-for-cup for the unbleached and whole-wheat flours.

LUNCH

11. Homemade Einkorn Tortillas

Prep Time: 50 minutes

Cook Time: 60 Minutes

Yield: Servings 12 to 14 Tortillas

Ingredient

- 2-1/4 cups (280 g) all-purpose einkorn flour, plus up to 1/4 cup (31 g) more
- 1/4 cup (60 ml) olive oil or melted coconut oil (or a combination of the two)
- 1/4 teaspoon sea salt
- 1/2 cup (120 ml) warm water (100 to 110 degrees F [37 to 43 C])

Instructions

1. In a medium-size bowl, stir together flour, olive oil, salt, and warm water. Using clean hands, work the mixture together into a ball of dough, kneading it in

the bowl until it comes together. Set the ball in the bowl and cover with a towel; let rest for 15 to 30 minutes.

2. On a floured surface or large piece of parchment paper, divide the dough into 12 to 14 balls, each about 1-1/2-inches (3.8 cm) wide.

3. Heat a cast iron skillet over medium heat on the stove. If using a tortilla press, line both sides of the press with plastic wrap, and flatten 1 dough round between the press. If not using a tortilla press, use a rolling pin and a floured surface to roll 1 dough round into a 5 to 6-inch (13 to 15 cm) circle.

4. Working with one at a time, place a flattened tortilla on the hot skillet. Within a minute or two, you should start seeing a lot of bubbles forming on the top of the dough. At this point, use kitchen tongs or a spatula to flip the tortilla and cook for right around a minute on the other side, until both sides are golden, with brown spots, and firm. Remove tortilla to a clean towel and cover to keep warm. Repeat rolling and cooking process with remaining dough.

Prep Time: 55 minutes

Cook Time: 35 Minutes

Yield: Servings 4

Ingredient

- 2 red bell peppers
- 1 pound fingerling potatoes
- 1-1/5 pounds sweet potato, cut into 1-inch pieces
- Salt
- 2 (5-ounce) cans waterpacked U.S. albacore tuna, water drained and reserved
- 6 ounces slivered almonds, toasted
- 3 tablespoons Classic Aioli or mayonnaise
- 2 tablespoons extra-virgin olive oil
- 1 teaspoon freshly grated nutmeg, for garnish

Instructions

1. Roast the peppers directly over the burners of a gas stove or under the broiler until the skins are blackened all over.

2. Remove from the heat and place in a loosely sealed bag to steam.

3. Taking care to save any juices, peel the peppers (it's okay to leave some black flecks or small patches of skin). Remove and discard the seeds, then cut the peppers into thin strips.

4. Meanwhile, place the fingerlings and sweet potatoes in a pan with a generous pinch of salt and the reserved tuna water, cover with cold water, and cook until they can be easily pierced with a knife, about 10 minutes.

5. Drain the potatoes, then toss gently with the almonds, aioli, reserved pepper juices, and olive oil to combine.

6. Arrange the potato mixture on a platter and top with the pepper strips and any juices.

7. Gently flake the tuna and scatter it over the salad. Sprinkle the nutmeg over the salad and serve.

Prep Time: 20 minutes

Cook Time: 45 Minutes

Yield: Servings 4

Ingredient

- 1 small cauliflower, broken into small florets
- 1 little gem lettuce
- 5 to 6 cherry tomatoes, halved
- 1/3 large cucumber, peeled, seeded, and cut into half moons
- 5 to 6 radishes, coarsely chopped
- 2 pitas, toasted
- 2 tablespoons fresh flat-leaf parsley
- 2 tablespoons fresh cilantro
- 1 tablespoon fresh mint
- sea salt and freshly ground black pepper

For The Cauliflower Marinade:

- 1 teaspoon smoked paprika, plus extra to serve
- 1 teaspoon ground cumin
- 1/2 teaspoon ground cinnamon

- 1/2 teaspoon chile powder
- 1/2 teaspoon allspice
- pinch of cayenne pepper
- juice of 1/2 lime
- 1 teaspoon agave nectar
- 1/2 tablespoon olive oil

For The Chile Salad Dressing:

- 1 teaspoon chile paste from a jar
- 1 tablespoon red wine vinegar
- 1 teaspoon agave nectar
- juice of 1/2 lime
- 3 tablespoons olive oil

For The Tahini Dressing:

- 3 tablespoons hummus
- 2 tablespoons tahini
- 1 teaspoon agave nectar
- juice of 1/2 lime

Instructions

1. Preheat the oven to 400 degrees Fahrenheit. Place the cauliflower florets in a baking dish. Whisk the

marinade ingredients together, along with some seasoning, to form a smooth paste and pour over the cauliflower florets. Toss together until everything is coated and bake for about 45 minutes or until nicely browned. 2. Put the lettuce, tomatoes, cucumber, and radishes in a large bowl. Whisk the chile dressing ingredients together and pour about one-third over the salad. Mix together. Lightly toast or grill the pitas and cut into triangular bite-sized pieces. Drizzle over about one third of the chile dressing and add to the salad bowl. 4. Finely chop the parsley, cilantro, and mint together on a clean cutting board and sprinkle two thirds over the salad bowl ingredients. Gently mix.

2. Whisk the tahini sauce ingredients together with 1/4 cup water until smooth, adding more water if necessary.

3. Remove the roasted cauliflower from the oven and lightly season with some sea salt. Add to the salad and gently toss. Serve in a bowl, drizzle with the tahini dressing and a smattering of smoked paprika, and garnish with the remaining parsley, cilantro, and mint.

Prep Time: 20 minutes

Cook Time: 45 Minutes

Yield: Servings 4

Ingredient

- 2 lbs (1 kg) boneless, skinless chicken breasts, diced
- 1/2 tsp (2 mL) garlic salt
- 2 tbsp (30 mL) vegetable oil
- 1 onion, quartered
- 1 tbsp (15 mL) minced garlic
- 1 tsp (5 mL) minced or grated fresh ginger
- 1/2 jalapeño pepper
- 2 cans (each 14 oz/398 mL) coconut milk
- 2 cups (500 mL) chicken broth or Homemade Chicken Stock
- 2 tbsp (30 mL) curry powder
- 1 tsp (5 mL) salt
- 1/4 tsp (1 mL) freshly ground black pepper
- 1-1/2 tsp (7 mL) dried basil
- 1/2 cup (125 mL) salted roasted cashews

Instructions

1. Sprinkle chicken with garlic salt. In a large wok or skillet over high heat, heat vegetable oil until smoking. Working in batches, add chicken and cook for 3 to 4 minutes, stirring constantly, until no longer pink inside and slightly crispy on one or two edges. Using a slotted spoon, transfer chicken to a bowl and set aside.

2. In a blender or food processor, combine onion, garlic, ginger and jalapeño; blend on high until smooth. Add coconut milk, chicken broth, curry powder, salt and pepper; blend until smooth. In a large saucepan, combine chicken and any accumulated juices, coconut milk mixture and dried basil. Bring to a boil over medium-high heat. Immediately reduce heat to low and simmer for 15 minutes to deepen flavors. Remove from heat. Ladle into bowls and top with cashews, plus cilantro, fresh basil and jalapeño, if using. Make It a Freezer Meal Let chicken cool completely. Pour chicken, coconut milk mixture and dried basil into a labeled gallon-size freezer bag. Seal, removing as much air as possible, and freeze. Place cashews in a quart-size freezer bag and seal. Place both bags in another gallon bag and seal together. Place soup in

refrigerator for at least 12 hours or up to 24 hours to thaw, or run lukewarm water over bag until you can break soup apart. Pour bag contents into a large saucepan and bring to a boil over medium-high heat. Immediately reduce heat to low and simmer for 15 minutes to deepen flavors. Remove from heat. Ladle into bowls and top with cashews, plus cilantro, fresh basil and jalapeño, if using is an urban homesteader wannabe.

Prep Time: 40 minutes

Cook Time: 50 Minutes

Yield: Servings 6

Ingredient

- 1/4 cup (60 mL) melted butter
- 1/4 cup (60 mL) chicken broth
- Grated zest and juice of 2 large lemons
- 1-1/2 tsp (7 mL) dried dill
- 1/2 tsp (2 mL) minced garlic
- 2 lbs (1 kg) skinless tilapia fillets (about six 6 oz/175 g pieces)

To serve:

- 2 tbsp (30 mL) olive oil
- 12 6-inch (15 cm) corn tortillas, warmed
- Toppings
- cup (250 mL) shredded lettuce
- 1 cup (250 mL) canned or cooked black beans, drained and rinsed (optional)
- 1/4 cup (60 mL) salsa or pico de gallo (optional)

Instructions

1. In a small bowl, whisk together melted butter, chicken broth, lemon zest, lemon juice, dill and garlic.

2. Place marinade mixture and tilapia fillets in a gallon-size (4 L) freezer bag or bowl. (Label the bag if freezing for later.) Seal bag, removing as much air as possible, or cover bowl. Transfer to refrigerator to marinate for 15 minutes. Preheat oven to 400 degrees. Drizzle olive oil over a rimmed baking sheet. Transfer baking sheet to oven while it preheats. Once oven is preheated, remove baking sheet from oven, add fillets and return it to oven. Bake for 10 to 12 minutes, until fish is flaky and lightly crisped on the edges. Remove from oven and chop into chunks. Arrange tortillas on a work surface. Evenly divide fish and lettuce, plus beans and salsa (if using), among tortillas. Serve. Make It a Freezer Meal Freeze bag. Place bag in the refrigerator for 12 to 24 hours to thaw. Preheat oven to 400 degrees. (Drizzle olive oil over a rimmed baking sheet. Transfer baking sheet to oven while it preheats. Once oven is preheated, remove baking sheet from oven, add fillets and return it to oven. Bake for 10 to 12 minutes, until fish is flaky and lightly crisped on the edges. Remove from oven

and chop into chunks. Arrange tortillas on a work surface. Evenly divide fish and lettuce, plus beans and salsa, if using, among tortillas. Serve.

Prep Time: 52 minutes

Cook Time: 55 Minutes

Yield: Servings 6

Ingredient

- 1 1/4 cups vegetable stock
- 1/2 cup dried giant wholewheat couscous
- small handful of flat-leaf parsley, chopped
- 9 oz heritage carrots (I particularly love purple ones)
- few thyme sprigs, leaves picked
- 1/2 tsp cumin seeds
- grated zest of 1 orange
- 3 tbsp olive oil
- 3 tbsp plain yogurt
- grated zest and juice of 1/2 lemon
- 1 garlic clove, very finely chopped
- sea salt and freshly ground black pepper
- small handful of rocket (arugula)
- scant 1/4 cup golden sultanas (golden raisins)

Instructions

1. Preheat the oven to 325 degrees Fahrenheit.

2. Bring the stock to the boil in a pan, then add the couscous. Cover with a lid, reduce the heat and simmer for about 6 minutes, or until the couscous is soft but still with a bite.

3. Remove from the heat and leave to cool. When the couscous is cool, fold through the chopped parsley, then set aside in the pan.

4. While the couscous is cooling, cut the carrots into long sticks and toss in the thyme, cumin, orange zest and 2 tbsp olive oil. Place them on a baking tray and roast in the hot oven for 20–30 minutes until tender. When done, stir the roasted carrots into the couscous with all the roasting juices.

5. To make the dressing, mix the yogurt, lemon, remaining olive oil and garlic with some seasoning in a small jar and keep refrigerated until serving – just don't forget it in the morning!

6. Start filling your jar with the couscous and carrots, followed by the rocket and sultanas.

7. Add the dressing in lovely dollops and mix it up a bit for maximum flavor.

Prep Time: 10 minutes

Cook Time: 25 Minutes

Yield: Servings 6

Ingredient

- 1 roughly chopped zucchini (about 4–5 ounces)
- 1/2 cup packed spinach, or one big handful
- 2 large eggs
- 2/3 teaspoon sea salt
- 1 tablespoon lemon juice
- 1 tablespoon coconut flour
- 1 tablespoon psyllium husk powder

Instructions

1. Preheat your oven to 350°F.
2. Blend everything except the psyllium husk powder and coconut flour in your blender until nice and smooth and pour into a bowl.
3. Stir together the coconut flour and psyllium husk, whisk into the batter, and let rest a minute.

4. Use a baking liner or lightly butter or oil a cookie sheet and measure two portions of batter onto a baking sheet.

5. Use an offset spatula to spread batter into thin wraps.

6. Bake for about 10–12 minutes.

7. If you use two cookie sheets, you can bake four tortillas at once, on two even racks.

Prep Time: 25 minutes

Cook Time: 55 Minutes

Yield: Servings 3

Ingredient

- 3/4 cup red quinoa, rinsed very well
- 1-1/2 cups filtered or spring water
- 1 can (15 ounces) chickpeas (garbanzo beans), drained and rinsed
- 2 tablespoons extra-virgin olive oil
- 4 tablespoons freshly squeezed lemon juice
- 1 small red onion, diced
- 1 large clove garlic, minced
- 1 teaspoon Italian seasoning
- 1/4 teaspoon sea salt, plus more as needed
- 1/8 teaspoon cayenne pepper
- 1/8 teaspoon freshly ground pepper, plus more as needed
- 1 cup chopped fresh flat-leaf parsley
- 1/2 cup sweet red pepper, diced
- 2 medium avocados

Instructions

1. Put the quinoa and water in a medium sauce pan and bring to a boil over medium heat. Decrease the heat to medium-low, cover, and simmer for 15 to 18 minutes until all of the liquid is absorbed and the quinoa is soft.

2. Meanwhile, place the chickpeas, 1 tablespoon olive oil, 1 tablespoon lemon juice, onion, garlic, Italian seasoning, salt, cayenne pepper, and pepper in a large mixing bowl. Let the bean mixture stand at room temperature for about 20 minutes.

3. Put the cooked quinoa in a medium bowl. Toss with 1 tablespoon lemon juice and 1 tablespoon olive oil while it is still warm. Let the quinoa mixture cool for about 15 minutes.

4. Add the quinoa to the chickpea mixture. Add the parsley, red pepper, and remaining lemon juice. Stir gently to combine. Cover and refrigerate for 2 hours.

5. Right before serving, cube the avocados and add them to the salad. Toss gently to combine. Serve over lettuce leaves with whole-grain bread on the side. Season with additional salt and pepper.

6.

Prep Time: 25 minutes

Cook Time: 55 Minutes

Yield: Servings 6

Ingredient

- 6 stalks celery, with leaves, chopped
- 1 sweet onion, chopped
- 1 teaspoon Italian seasoning or other herb blend
- 8 cups vegetable broth
- 1 teaspoon reduced-sodium tamari
- 3 cups water, plus more as needed
- 2 medium sweet potatoes, peeled and chopped
- 5 medium red potatoes, peeled and chopped
- 5 carrots, chopped
- 2 cups chopped green beans
- 6 large cremini or white button mushrooms, sliced
- 1 can (15 ounces) white beans, drained and rinsed
- Sea salt
- Freshly ground pepper

Instructions

1. Put the celery, onion, Italian seasoning, and 1/4 cup of the broth in a large soup pot over medium heat. Cook, stirring occasionally, until the onion is translucent, about 8 minutes, adding more broth as needed, 1 tablespoon at a time, if the mixture becomes dry.

2. Stir in the tamari and cook, stirring occasionally, until the celery and onion are tender, about 8 minutes.

3. Stir in the remaining broth, the water, sweet potatoes, red potatoes, carrots, green beans, and mushrooms. Decrease the heat, cover, and simmer, stirring occasionally, for 30 minutes.

4. Stir in the white beans and simmer until the vegetables are tender, 15 to 20 minutes longer, adding more water as needed to achieve the desired consistency. Season with salt and pepper to taste. Serve piping hot.

Prep Time: 25 minutes

Cook Time: 55 Minutes

Yield: Servings 6

Ingredient

Taco Bowls:

- 4 8- to 10-inch whole-grain tortillas (spicy variety works well)

Salad:

- 2 large ripe avocados
- 2 tablespoons freshly squeezed lemon juice
- 1 teaspoon chili powder
- 1/4 teaspoon ground turmeric
- 1/4 teaspoon smoked paprika
- 1/4 teaspoon sea salt, plus more as needed
- 1/16 to 1/8 teaspoon cayenne pepper (optional)
- 1 medium tomato, diced
- 1/2 medium sweet onion, diced
- 2-1/2 cups thinly sliced romaine lettuce

- 1/4 cup chopped fresh parsley or cilantro, for garnish (optional)
- Zest of one lemon, for garnish (optional)

Instructions

1. Preheat the oven to 400 degrees F. Line a medium, rimmed baking pan with unbleached parchment paper.

2. Arrange four small oven-safe bowls upside down on the prepared pan. Drape a tortilla over the bottom of each bowl, arranging it in the shape of an upside-down "bowl." Bake for 10 to 15 minutes, or until the tortillas are crisp and almost firm to the touch, checking them often so they do not burn. Carefully transfer the pan with the bowls on it to a wire rack and let cool at least 5 minutes before serving.

3. Meanwhile, to prepare the guacamole, peel, pit and rough chop the avocados. Put the chopped avocados, lemon juice, chili powder, turmeric, smoked paprika, sea salt and cayenne pepper (optional) in a medium-sized bowl and mash with a potato masher or large fork until combined. Gently fold in the tomatoes and onion.

4. To assemble the salads, carefully remove each cooled taco "bowl" and place it in the center of a medium-sized salad plate. Place one-quarter of the sliced romaine in the bottom of each taco "bowl." Top with one-quarter of the guacamole mixture. Garnish with a sprinkle of chopped fresh parsley or cilantro, and lemon zest (optional). Serve immediately.

Prep Time: 15 minutes

Cook Time: 45 Minutes

Yield: Servings 4

Ingredient

- 4 tablespoons golden flaxseeds
- 2 large ripe bananas
- 1/4 cup Sucanat, brown sugar, or your preferred dry sweetener
- 2 heaping tablespoons blueberry preserves
- 1 teaspoon vanilla extract
- 2 cups rolled oats
- 1/4 cup raw unsweetened shredded dried coconut
- 1 cup fresh blueberries

Instructions

1. Preheat the oven to 375 degrees F. Line an 8-inch square baking pan with unbleached parchment paper, leaving 3- to 4-inch "wings" on two opposite sides of the pan.

2. Put the flaxseeds in a high-performance blending appliance and process into very fine flour. Put the bananas, Sucanat (or brown sugar), blueberry preserves and vanilla in a medium-sized bowl and mash with a potato masher or large fork into a chunky purée. Add the ground flaxseeds, oats and coconut; stir to combine. Gently fold in the fresh blueberries.

3. Spread the dough in an even layer in the prepared pan. Score into 10 bars using a table knife. Bake for 30 to 35 minutes, or until slightly golden around the edges. Put the pan on a heatproof surface. Using the parchment paper "wings" as handles, carefully lift the bars out of the pan in one piece. Transfer to a wire rack and let cool for 15 to 20 minutes.

4. Again, using the parchment paper "wings" as handles, transfer the bars to a cutting board and cut into 10 individual bars. Stored in an airtight container in the refrigerator, the bars will keep for 2 days.

5. 145 Calories; 3g Fat; 1g Saturated fat; 3g Protein; 6mg Sodium; 29g Total Carbohydrate; 12g Sugars; 4g Fiber

DINNER

21. Chicken in Wine with Mushrooms, Peas, and Herbs

Prep Time: 35 minutes

Cook Time: 50 Minutes

Yield: Servings 3

Ingredient

- 1 whole chicken, about 4 pounds, cut into pieces
- 2 tablespoons butter
- 2 leeks, thinly sliced
- 1 pound button mushrooms, thinly sliced
- 1 teaspoon finely ground sea salt
- 2 cups dry white wine
- 1-1/2 pounds English peas in their shell, or 2 cups frozen peas
- 1 bunch flat-leaf parsley, finely chopped
- 1 bunch chives, finely chopped
- 1/2 cup crème fraiche

Instructions

1. Warm the butter in the bottom of a Dutch oven over medium heat.

2. Working in batches to prevent overcrowding, add the chicken pieces to the pot and brown them, about 6 minutes on each side.

3. Remove the chicken from the pan and stir then stir in the leeks and mushrooms. Add the salt to the pot, cover it, and turn down the heat to medium-low.

4. Allow the leeks and mushrooms to sweat together in the heat of the pot until tender, about 8 minutes.

5. Return the chicken to the pot and then pour in the white wine.

6. Simmer it all together over medium-low heat until the chicken is tender, about 45 minutes. If you're using fresh peas still in their shell, shell them while the chicken cooks. Pour them into the pan and then continue simmering them all together until the peas soften and become tender, a further 20 minutes. If you're using frozen peas, continue cooking the chicken another 15 minutes and then pour in the peas, allowing them to warm, about 5 minutes more. Stir the parsley and chives into the pot. Turn off the heat,

stir in the crème fraîche, season with sea salt, and
serve hot.

Prep Time: 25 minutes

Cook Time: 60 Minutes

Yield: Servings 6

Ingredient

- 3 tablespoons extra virgin olive oil, divided, plus more to form patties
- 1 yellow onion, sliced into 1/4-inch-thick rounds
- 2 garlic cloves, roughly chopped
- 1 cup Spiced Black Beans
- 1-1/2 cups Cumin-Roasted Sweet Potatoes
- 1 tablespoon Worcestershire sauce
- 1/2 teaspoon sea salt
- 1 teaspoon smoked paprika
- 1 teaspoon chili powder
- 1 teaspoon ground cumin
- 1-1/2 cups Green Rice
- 1/3 cup panko bread crumbs
- 4 to 6 toasted whole-wheat or sprouted-grain buns

Optional Garnishes:

- 1 avocado, peeled, pitted and sliced
- 1 bunch arugula or microgreens
- 1 small jar sliced pickled beets or sun-dried tomatoes
- Mayonnaise, mustard and ketchup

Instructions

1. In a large skillet over medium heat, warm 2 tablespoons olive oil until shimmering, and add onion rounds. Sauté until fragrant and beginning to caramelize, about 15 minutes. Stir every few minutes to avoid sticking. Add a little bit of water and reduce heat to low if onions begin to color too quickly before softening.
2. Reduce heat and add garlic. Stir well and cook for another minute.
3. In the bowl of a food processor, add onion-garlic mixture, beans, sweet potatoes, Worcestershire sauce, salt and spices. Pulse to form a thick, chunky puree. Spoon mixture out into a large bowl, fold in rice and stir to combine thoroughly. Cover and refrigerate mixture for at least 1 hour and up to 3 days.

4. Remove mixture from fridge. Lightly oil your hands and divide mixture into 4 or 6 equal portions. Shape each into patties about 1-inch-thick.

5. Heat remaining 1 tablespoon oil in a large skillet over medium heat and set patties into skillet (you'll likely only be able to cook 3 to 4 at a time, depending on size of skillet). Cook patty on each side for about 4 to 6 minutes, or until golden brown. Add a little more oil to the pan if they begin to stick. Serve on buns with desired garnishes and condiments.

Prep Time: 25 minutes

Cook Time: 60 Minutes

Yield: Servings 6

Ingredient

Potatoes:

- 1-1/2 pounds new potatoes, quartered or cut into eighths
- 2 tablespoons extra-virgin olive oil
- 3 garlic cloves, minced
- 2 teaspoons fresh thyme leaves, or 1 teaspoon dried
- Salt and freshly ground black pepper

Chicken and Artichokes:

- 2 tablespoons extra-virgin olive oil
- 1 pound boneless, skinless chicken breasts, cut into bite-size pieces
- Salt and freshly ground black pepper
- 2 cans (14 ounces each) artichoke hearts, quartered and drained
- 1/2 cup chicken broth

- 2 tablespoons fresh lemon juice
- 1/4 cup chopped fresh parsley
- 1/2 cup pitted, brine-cured black olives, such as kalamata, chopped

Instructions

Potatoes:

1. Preheat the oven to 425 degrees Fahrenheit.
2. Lightly oil a large sheet pan.
3. Combine the potatoes, oil, garlic, thyme, and salt and pepper to taste in a bowl. Toss well.
4. Spread out the potatoes on the sheet pan in a single layer.
5. Roast for 25 minutes, until browned all over, shaking the pan occasionally for even cooking. Set aside.

Chicken and Artichokes:

1. Heat the oil in a large skillet over medium-high heat.
2. Sauté the chicken in the oil until white and firm, 6 to 8 minutes. Season to taste with salt and pepper.
3. Add the artichoke hearts, chicken broth, and lemon juice to the skillet. Cook until the liquid in the pan reduces and is slightly thickened, about 2 minutes.

4. Mix in the potatoes. Garnish with the parsley and
   olives. Serve at once.

Prep Time: 55 minutes

Cook Time: 60 Minutes

Yield: Servings 3

Ingredient

- 1 10-inch whole-grain sandwich wrap or tortilla
- 2 to 3 tablespoons low-fat prepared marinara sauce
- 1/4 teaspoon Italian seasoning blend
- 1/8 teaspoon crushed red pepper
- 2 cups lightly packed baby spinach, washed and dried
- 4 green queen olives with pimento, sliced (see note)
- 10 to 12 slices vegan pepperoni, or 4 very thinly sliced cremini mushrooms
- 1/3 cup shredded vegan cheese (optional)

Instructions

1. Preheat the oven to 400 degrees F.
2. Put the sandwich wrap on a large baking sheet or pizza pan. Spread the marinara sauce over the wrap, in an even layer, leaving a slight margin around the

edge for a "crust." Sprinkle the Italian seasoning and crushed pepper over the sauce. Top with the baby spinach, pressing it down to make it more compact.

3. Top with the olives, vegan pepperoni (or mushrooms) and vegan cheese (optional). Bake for 10 to 12 minutes or until crust is crisp and toppings are heated through. Cut into wedges and serve.

Prep Time: 15 minutes

Cook Time: 40 Minutes

Yield: Servings 3

Ingredient

- 3/4 cup (150g) cooked white rice
- 2 large eggs
- salt and pepper (use white pepper if you want the omelets without black specks)
- olive oil for frying
- 1/4 medium onion, chopped
- 1/4 large red bell pepper, chopped
- 1 teaspoon butter
- 2 oz (60g) cooked chicken, chopped
- 2 tablespoons ketchup, for the rice
- ketchup for decoration, optional

Instructions

1. If you are using pre-frozen rice, defrost it before using.

2. Beat the eggs with a pinch of salt and pepper.

3. Heat a little olive oil in a nonstick frying pan over medium heat. Put in the onion and sauté until it starts to turn translucent. Add the chopped bell pepper and sauté until softened. Add the rice and butter, and sauté until the rice is well coated with oil and butter. Add the chicken and ketchup, and mix well. Season with salt and pepper.

4. Remove the rice from the pan and wipe the pan out with a paper towel. Add a little more oil and heat the pan over high heat. When the pan is hot, add the eggs and spread it around rapidly. Turn the heat down to low, and leave the eggs to cook through completely. Remove from the heat until ready to pack.

Prep Time: 15 minutes

Cook Time: 50 Minutes

Yield: Servings 3

Ingredient

- -1/2 pounds red potatoes, quartered or cut into eighths
- 3 tablespoons extra-virgin olive oil 3 garlic cloves, minced 1 teaspoon dried oregano Salt and freshly ground black pepper 1/2 pound sweet or hot Italian sausage, sliced 1 inch thick 1 onion, halved and slivered 8 cups chopped fresh kale, tough stems discarded 1-1/2 cups chicken broth 1 can (15 ounces) cannellini beans, rinsed and drained

Instructions

1. Preheat the oven to 425 degrees F. Lightly grease a large baking sheet with oil.
2. Combine the potatoes, 2 tablespoons of the oil, garlic, oregano, and salt and pepper to taste in a medium

bowl and toss to coat. Spread out in a single layer on the baking sheet and roast for about 25 minutes, until browned and tender.

3. Heat the remaining 1 tablespoon oil in a large skillet. Sauté the sausage and onion in the oil until the sausage is mostly browned, 4 to 6 minutes.

4. Stir in half the kale and all the broth. Cook, stirring, until the kale is wilted. Stir in the remaining kale. Cover and simmer for about 5 minutes, until the kale is wilted and tender but still bright green.

5. Mix in the beans, then the potatoes, Season with salt and pepper and serve at once.

Prep Time: 15 minutes

Cook Time: 50 Minutes

Yield: Servings 3

Ingredient

- 1-1/4 cups, about 6 oz sweet potato, grated
- 1/2 red onion, finely sliced
- 2 cloves garlic, crushed
- 1 teaspoon fennel seeds
- 2 tablespoon coconut oil
- 1/2 teaspoon sunflower oil

To serve

- 1 cup spinach, wilted
- 4 eggs poached or 1/2 cup goat cheese if you prefer

Instructions

1. I find it best to make the rosti in batches, 2 at a time, so you will need to repeat the following process twice.

2. Put the grated sweet potato into a cloth or dish towel and squeeze all the excess water out: you want the pulp to be as dry as possible. Transfer to a bowl.

3. Melt half the coconut oil in a non-stick pan and sauté half of the red onion, garlic and fennel seeds for 1 minute. Add half the sweet potato and stir continuously for 30 seconds, so that the potato absorbs all the other flavors. Transfer to the bowl containing the remaining sweet potato and mix well.

4. Wipe the frying pan clean and spread half the oil around it with a cloth or paper towel. Place over medium heat.

5. Divide the rosti mixture into 4 equal pieces and form into patties. Place 2 of them in the hot pan and press down slightly. Cook for about 3-4 minutes on each side or until they are golden. Keep them warm while you cook the remaining patties in the same way.

6. When finished, set the patties aside while you repeat the process with the remaining mixture.

7. Serve with the spinach and poached eggs or goat cheese.

Prep Time: 15 minutes

Cook Time: 50 Minutes

Yield: Servings 3

Ingredient

- 1 small red cabbage (about 1-3/4 pounds)
- 1/4 cup mirin
- 1-1/2 teaspoons sea salt
- 1-1/2 teaspoons Chinese five-spice powder
- 2 tablespoons extra virgin olive oil
- 1 bunch green onions, white and green parts, thinly sliced
- 1/2 cup sliced almonds, toasted (see Cook's Note)
- 1 avocado, halved, pitted, peeled, diced and tossed with a large pinch of salt

Instructions

1. To chop cabbage, halve head through stem end, cut out core and place halves cut-side down. Cut halves into 1/4-inch-thick slices, then rotate the slices 90

degrees and cut across slices to create 1/4-inch pieces. You will have about 8 cups.

2. In a large bowl, toss cabbage with mirin, salt and five-spice powder. Let stand for 15 minutes at room temperature, or up to 2 hours in refrigerator if you plan to serve salad chilled.

3. Add oil, green onions and almonds, and toss. Taste and add additional salt and mirin if needed. Add avocado and toss gently. The salad will wilt; eat it within a few hours for optimum crunch.

29. Apple Brown Betty

Prep Time: 30 minutes

Cook Time: 45 Minutes

Yield: Servings 3

Ingredient

1 teaspoon cinnamon

1/4 cup brown sugar

2 slices sandwich bread cut in 1/4-inch cubes (I used honey whole wheat)

1 tablespoons melted butter

1 tablespoon lemon zest

3-4 cups apple slices (about 1lb) – no need to peel

2 tablespoons apple cider or water

Instructions

1. Preheat the oven to 375°F.
2. Combine the cinnamon and the sugar and set aside 2 tablespoons. Put the bread cubes in a bowl and toss

with the rest of the sugar mixture, the melted butter, and the lemon rind.

3. Line the bottom of a casserole with half of the bread cubes. Layer the apple slices over the bread and sprinkle with the cider or water. Top with the remaining bread cubes and sprinkle with the reserved 2 tablespoons of sugar. Cover the casserole and bake for 40 minutes, then remove the lid and bake an additional 10 to 15 minutes, or until apples are tender and the topping is brown.

4. Serve with ice cream or whipped cream for a special treat!

5. Serving a crowd? Double the recipe, use a larger casserole, and make with five layers instead of three. Easy-peasy!

Prep Time: 10 minutes

Cook Time: 30 Minutes

Yield: Servings 3

Ingredient

- 2 tablespoons extra-virgin olive oil
- 2 cups white mushrooms, sliced
- 1 onion, thinly sliced
- 1 green bell pepper, diced
- 3 large garlic cloves, minced
- 1 can (28 ounces) plum tomatoes with juice, chopped
- 4-5 cups chicken broth
- 1 tablespoon chopped fresh basil, or 1 teaspoon dried
- 1 teaspoon chopped fresh or dried rosemary
- 1 teaspoon chopped fresh thyme, or 1/2 teaspoon dried
- 1-1/2–2 cups cooked chicken, diced
- Salt and freshly ground black pepper

Instructions

1. Heat the oil in a large soup pot over medium-high heat. Sauté the mushrooms, onion, and green pepper in the oil for about 5 minutes, until the mushrooms begin to give up their juice. Add the garlic and sauté for another minute.

2. Add the tomatoes, broth, basil, rosemary, and thyme. Bring to a boil, then reduce the heat and simmer, uncovered, for 30 to 45 minutes, until the flavors have blended.

3. Add the chicken and heat through. Season to taste with salt and pepper. Serve hot.